It's Not Too Late!
A BABY BOOMER'S GUIDE TO FITNESS

By
Robert Bresloff CFT, FT, AFS

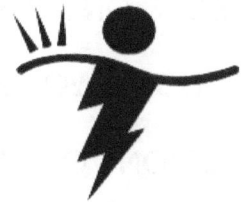

Copyright 2012

ISBN# 978-1-105-49539-7

It's Not Too Late! A Baby Boomers Guide to Fitness was written and prepared by Robert Bresloff. Robert is certified as a Personal Trainer, Fitness Therapist and Adaptive Fitness Specialist by International Sports Sciences Association. (ISSA)

It's Not Too Late!

TABLE OF CONTENTS

Photography—Joe Bresloff

It's Not Too Late!

PREFACE

We might not be getting any younger, but I can't think of one good reason not to meet those coming golden years head on. Exercise may or may not be the fountain of youth but having strong bones, supple, flexible muscles and great balance can make getting older a lot easier to take.

Every day we read more and about how our generation needs to deal with health issues such as osteoporosis, heart disease, diabetes, high blood pressure, chronic back problems and obesity. Make no mistake about it; fitness and health are two completely different issues but one can help the other. Proper fitness can positively affect many common health complaints.

Truly, we're not getting any younger and though being fit doesn't carry any guarantees, a well balanced fitness program can do wonders for the body and the mind. Attitude is everything. Remember we're all the same age. Some of us have just been here a little longer.

Over the last twenty years we have probably seen hundreds of new "innovations" in the fitness world as well as all the "Gurus" that have tried to sell us on the idea that only they can lead the way to the true "promised land" of fitness. It is because of these folks and their empty promises to our generation that I decided to write this book.

After many years of lifting weights, coaching sports and personal training (at this writing I am 62 years young and still a full-time personal trainer), I have come to realize that not only do most of these so called experts that we see on television, in books and magazines not have the answer, I don't even think they know the question!

There is so much more to fitness than glistening pecs and bulging biceps, especially at our age. The human body has a set of rules that it must live by— they're called biomechanics. Many of these so-called experts seem to ignore this fact and continually teach methods that could be injurious to joints. My hope is that this book will teach you proper exercises performed in a functional manner designed to get results while at the same time protecting your joints, leaving them strong, flexible and ready to meet the challenges of middle or any age. This exercise system is no quick fix and in no way does it pretend to have all the answers—but it **is** a well thought out plan that takes physical limitations into consideration.

Why in the world do we need to train in the martial arts style if we don't practice martial arts? Why do we take classes that make us step up and down on the same riser over and over again (without any regard to proper knee tracking or foot placement) when we should be teaching our bodies how to properly climb a **flight** of stairs? Don't even get me started on fitness boot camps.

After all these years, I have learned the significance of balance, stability, joint range and how to teach human beings to exercise properly without the pain, soreness and injuries that have come to be expected with working out.

Remember this one, "No Pain No Gain"? It even sounds ridiculous, doesn't it? On the following pages I will attempt to teach you proper form and the proper progression of exercise done correctly. Some of the theory you are about to experience may contradict popular beliefs but if you think it through, I'm sure that you will agree that it makes perfect, logical sense. Okay baby-boomers, now let's begin learning the proper exercise methods that will get you in shape to tackle the most difficult sport of all—everyday life—your everyday life.

It's Not Too Late!

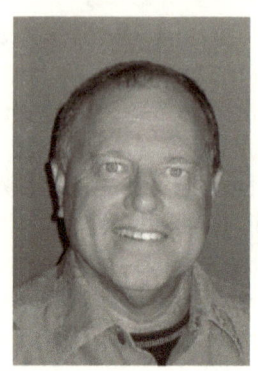

Robert Bresloff is a Certified Fitness Trainer, Adaptive Fitness Specialist and Fitness Therapist with Certifications from The Institute of Cellular Health and Fitness, International Sports Sciences Association, The Gajda Health Plus Network and The National Federation of Professional Trainers. Robert has spent over 25 years coaching sports and fitness.

It's Not Too Late!

SECTION ONE

Some Facts About Aging

The average human life expectancy is constantly changing. Once upon a time, back in the early 1900's, a human being was expected to only live to be 47 years of age. If you're reading this book, you're probably older than that now. Life was harder then. Most people worked at hard labor. It was a time when many people worked in factories or on the farm.

In 1900 the idea of proper nutrition was non existent. You pretty much ate what was available. Adequate medications for then common diseases were yet to come. Winters were colder (no I'm not referring to global warming; I'm talking about no central heating. Brrrr) and summers were hotter because there were no air-conditioners or electric fans to protect us from the heat. Face it, our live are a lot easier now.

So let's take another look at life expectancy. This time, we'll look at the 1990's. By this time a human being could expect to live around 75 years—big difference. (I guess those TV dinners weren't as bad for us as we thought).

A lot of things factor into this equation, but probably none so much as the advances made in modern medicine and nutrition.

It's Not Too Late!

These two factors alone are most responsible for the steady surge from 47 years in the early nineteen hundreds to 75 years at the end of the same century. Remember, fitness really didn't emerge as a force in aging until the late 1970's and by that time the average life expectancy was already well on the rise.

In the last fifteen to twenty years, hearing about someone celebrating their 70th birthday has become commonplace. Most people nowadays assume, barring any accidents or an unexpected illness that they will surely live that long and longer. As I said, it wasn't always so. As a people, Americans are growing older. But, will we be healthy when we reach seventy? Do older Americans reap the health benefits of exercise? Here are some interesting facts regarding aging and exercise.

As people age, their activity levels tend to drop. By age 75, three out of five aging adults have ceased participation in any type of physical activity. These aging adults have a higher risk factor of heart disease, high blood pressure, colon cancer and diabetes. Think about it. With as little as twenty minutes of exercise only three days a week it's possible to reduce the risk of these diseases. Sounds easy, huh?

As I said earlier, fitness offers no 'money back' guarantees and to exercise properly takes a lot of hard work. But, the possible rewards—stronger bones and muscles, increased circulation, fat loss, and reduced LDL cholesterol levels—can be there. Add a proper nutrition plan and who knows where exercise can take you.

Obesity is on the rise and osteoporosis is becoming more and more common. Unfortunately, both these problems are worsened by a sedentary life style. Without exercise aging Americans can become 'fat' and 'fragile'. The other unfortunate thing is that, as baby-boomers, we're at the age where an 'unhealthy lifestyle' is about to catch up with us.

That brings us to biomarkers. Biomarker is a relatively new term for the signs most associated by aging such as: slowing metabolism, (*Caloric requirements drop by 2-10 percent each decade over the age of 30), decrease in lean muscle mass, bone mass, cardiac output declines, decreasing aerobic capacity (Do you huff and puff climbing up stairs?), blood cholesterol levels rise, frequent urination (Guys, when was the last time you had a full nights sleep?). Do you want me to keep going?

Bottom line is, if you haven't yet experienced any of these changes you still have a chance to slow things down and enjoy a few more years without them. The truth is that human physiology changes as the years pile up. There's no way to avoid it. We will all eventually succumb to one, some or all of the conditions listed above.

Here's the funny thing, biomarkers can also be associated with a sedentary lifestyle at any adult age. I'm sure that we've all known someone in their thirties that was horribly out of shape. Chances are that person may have suffered from one or more of the aforementioned biomarkers. But at thirty, why not? A de-conditioned body is a de-conditioned body at any age.

On the next few pages, we will discuss the positive effects of *proper exercise* on aging. Read on baby-boomers, this is where it gets **really** interesting.

Proper Exercise and Its Possible Effects on Aging

Myths, myths, myths, they're everywhere. On TV, radio, newspapers and believe it or not, they're even at the place where you work out. Make no **myth**stake…sorry, I couldn't resist. Seriously, I'm sure you've watched an infomercial and turned to your wife, husband or friend and said, "Do you think that really works?"

Believe me it doesn't. Most of the myths that are out there such as: lying leg lifts really build strong abs, overhead shoulder presses are safe, the bench press is the only way to get strong Pecs and walking lunges really tighten the glutes. I'm sure that you've heard at least one of these.

The most overlooked and arguably the most important word in fitness is 'balance'. Why? Because this one word says it all—balance! We spend our entire lives trying to keep things in balance, our check book, our diet or time with family. We even make time for hobbies, all to 'balance' our time with our work.

Well, fitness is the same way. We need to 'balance' our work outs. You're probably wondering where this is going and a number of ideas have probably already crossed your mind. Things you might have heard at the gym or on TV.

Wrong! The kind of 'balance' I'm referring to is **muscle balance.** It is very important to make sure that any one muscle group does not overpower its opposing group.

People have a tendency to work harder on what they can easily see and neglect what they can't. I call this 'gym rat training' because every health club has a core group of folks that practically live there, constantly doing bench presses, bicep curls and leg extensions. You know who I'm talking about. This type of training easily affects everyone in the gym because, mistakenly, the casual exerciser believes that these, muscular guys and gals actually know what they're doing. Why not? They look great.

Next time you're at your club take a real close look at these guys (and gals. believe me, they're there as well). Don't stare. (I don't want anyone to get punched in the nose. A simple glance will do.) What do you see? Horribly rounded shoulders, terrible posture? That they're constantly, rotating or rubbing their joints after a lift? My guess is that you will answer yes to all of the above.

To get the most out of exercise, one must always keep in mind that everyday life is exercise too. What your occupation, hobby or physical activity may be does make a difference. If your job sits you in front of a computer all day, you may find that push exercises will come easier than pull. If you cycle, you have probably overdeveloped your quadriceps. If you kayak or crew you could have overdeveloped back muscles. Do you see where this is going?

We live in a push world. What that means is, on a daily basis we will probably use our pectorals (chest muscles) and anterior deltoids (front shoulder muscles) more than our rhomboids (middle back muscles that assist in pulling movements). That brings us to 'balance' again or in this case 'imbalance'.

Let's refer to stronger or more developed muscle groups as 'facilitated' and the weaker less developed ones as inhibited. In many cases, a person with a highly pronounced 'facilitation' of a certain muscle group should not need to exercise that muscle group until the opposing inhibited group is strong enough to balance.

Most of you have been in a health club. What do most clubs feature? Their 'high tech' exercise machines. Don't get me wrong, I think these machines can be very useful in making you stronger, but some problems do exist.

Let's take a look at these 'high tech' machines. There are usually one or more machines for every muscle group (most clubs have two each of the machines that work the facilitated muscles we discussed above—two pectorals quadriceps and bicep machines). Why? Because, they are usually the most popular machines in the club and people will complain when they can't get on them. Remember what I said earlier? People work most what people can see. If you continue to work already facilitated muscles, they will only get stronger at the expense of their much weaker opposing muscle.

If an excessive muscle imbalance exists working on the entire circuit of these machines will only make it worse. If you believe that this is the case, and that an imbalance may exist, I recommend making an appointment with a fitness specialist (be sure to ask for education, certification and years of experience) or a licensed physical therapist.

Here are a few things to look for: Rounded shoulders, toes pointing toward two and ten o'clock when you walk, not being able to lock your knees without great difficulty or discomfort and constant lower back pain.

If you feel that you do not have any type of pronounced muscle imbalance then the exercise program in this book should work for you. The system takes 'normal', common muscle balance into consideration and if followed correctly it should balance your muscles out. At the very least, you will get stronger in a safe and effective manner without increasing those imbalances.

The movements in this book can be performed with either free weights, pulley machines, body weight, bands or tubing. Many of the tubing exercises can be performed on standard health club pulley equipment. Don't be afraid to experiment. Remember; always err on the side of safety. Start with very light weights progressing slowly until you reach the prescribed rep range.

You will see, as you read on, that there is no chapter on cardiovascular exercise. Let's face it, if you're old enough to be reading a book on baby boomer fitness, I really don't recommend taking up running. Running or jogging is tough on the knees, feet and lower back. I most certainly do recommend brisk walking for one half hour at least three times a week. (It's most effective if you walk after your resistance work out, but walking on separate days is fine too). If you are already in a running program, in no way will this book try to stop you from doing something you enjoy. I'm just advocating that over-fifty isn't the best time to start running.

It's Not Too Late!

Introduction to the Exercises

In the workout chapters of this book we will help you perform exercises that work muscles related to actions in everyday life, in a safe and effective manner. As the book progresses so will you. In the Beginning workout we will teach you the basic exercises to train your "core", shoulders, and hips using proper form for the most effective workout. From there, we will slowly and safely take you to the Intermediate phase using the same techniques to challenge you and start showing results from your hard work. Next comes the Advanced phase of your training, here we will start using more difficult variations of exercises learned in the Beginning and Intermediate phases of the program. This is where the sky is the limit. But remember as you progress and as you get stronger you may have to purchase additional equipment or join a health club to perform at this level. As we go along, we will tell you what equipment you will need.

We will also address "reciprocal inhibition" and muscle resets so you can eliminate stretching. If the program is followed in the order given in each section, there is no need to stretch after your exercise session. We will cover that more in depth as we go along.

It's Not Too Late!

Thank you for giving this exercise system a try. Believe me, you won't be sorry. Let me help you get in shape the right way. So what are we waiting for Baby Boomers? Let's get started!

CAUTION: Anyone starting an exercise program for the first time should always check with their physician to see if they may have any problems that could be exacerbated by exercise. Your physician can outline any contraindications to specific exercises that would reduce the risk of worsening an existing condition.

Keep in mind that to achieve any reward such as improved fitness there is always a risk. There is a risk of after work out soreness or even injury. I have been very careful in preparing the programs at all levels to avoid this from happening, but we just want you to be prepared that these things can possibly happen.

On the following pages you will find the anatomy charts that show the muscles used in the exercise sheets. On those sheets you will find that some of the muscles are represented in solid white and others in solid black. The white represents the common inhibited or 'weak' muscles. The black show the common facilitated or 'strong' muscles.

These muscles are called out to illustrate how the human body can adjust to daily life. Certain muscles get stronger and others grow weaker as we go through everyday life. The muscles that we show in this section are considered the norm. In this book, we attempt to balance out your muscles naturally and safely.

If you have any questions about whether you have muscle imbalances, contact a reputable trainer in your area. If you feel any pain during any of the exercises or if you feel any joint pain at all, stop exercising and contact your physician immediately.

It's Not Too Late!

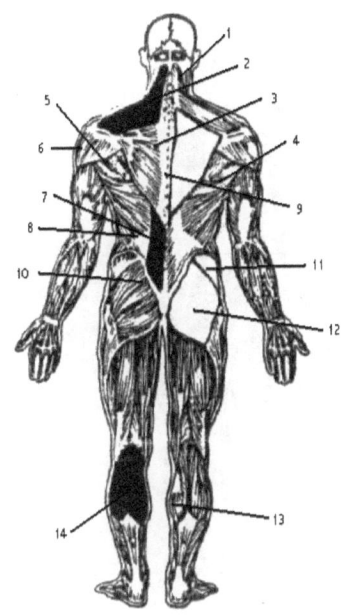

POSTERIOR VIEW

MUSCLES
1. Levator Scapulae
2. Upper Trapezius
3. Rhomboids (Deep)
4. Latissimus Dorsi
5. Teres Major
6. Posterior Deltoid
7. Lumbar Erector Spinae
8. Quadratus Lumborum (Deep)
9. Lower Middle Trapezius
10. Piriformis (Deep)
11. Gluteus Medius
12. Gluteus Maximus
13. Soleus
14. Gastrocnemius

It's Not Too Late!

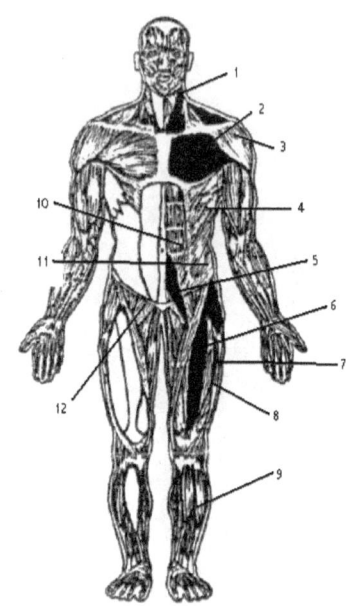

ANTERIOR VIEW

MUSCLES
1. Sternocleidomastoid
2. Pectoral Major & Minor
3. Anterior Deltoid
4. Serratus Anterior
5. PsoasMajor
6. Rectus Femoris
7. Tensor Fascia Latae (TFL)
8. Vasti Group (Quadraceps)
9. Anterior Tibialis
10. Rectus Abdominus
11. Obliques
12. Tranverse Abdominus

It's Not Too Late!

Before We Begin, A Word on Stretching

As we have illustrated in chapter one and two, the human body, over time, develops imbalances. For example, in most cases the pectorals are facilitated (strong) causing an inhibition (weakness) in the rhomboid (upper middle back) group. These imbalances take place throughout all the muscle groups; hamstrings (facilitated) and quadriceps (inhibited) is a good example.

My contention is that if a muscle group is already weak or flaccid what would be the benefit of stretching it. I believe the inhibited or weaker muscle should be worked after the facilitated or stronger muscle group. If the imbalance is pronounced, I will often suggest that a client refrain from working their facilitated group and train only the weaker group until balance is achieved. Again, if the muscles are long and weak, stretching is unnecessary it will only facilitate laxity (looseness) in the joint.

I have found little or no benefit from passive stretching. It will cause severe muscle imbalances by weakening an already inhibited muscle group. How often have you seen a runner pulling his heel to his glutes causing severe flexion to the knee? This can cause micro tears to the quadriceps group and laxity to the patella tendon and ligaments of the knee.

It's Not Too Late!

This has become an almost automatic stretch before and after running and is completely unnecessary. Quite often the muscular discomfort after an activity is from the micro-tears in the muscles caused by the stretching rather than the activity itself.

Do not automatically stretch before or after your workout. If you follow the order in which the exercises are given you should not feel the need to stretch. If you feel sore or feel that you need to stretch your muscles, please contact a fitness professional in your area to learn safe and proper techniques.

Remember, dogs and cats do not stretch. They use one muscle group to relax the opposing group. I bet you never saw a deer stretch either. Sometimes animals are smarter than people.

It's Not Too Late!

SECTION TWO

We Begin: The Equipment and How to Use It

Most pictures in this book illustrate the use of bands and tubing, but some of you may want to try some of these moves at your local gym or health club. Most of these clubs use machines that are restrictive and do not take rotation of the joints into consideration. They work the joints in a linear fashion, far from what actually happens in real life. Because of this, we recommend that you use free weights or pulley machines. You will see, as you learn the movements in our program that other than using tubes and bands, which are used in this book, pulleys will be the most efficient in performing, them.

It is very important that the equipment that you use, whether it is at your gym or in your home, be well maintained and in good working order. If there is any doubt that this is the case, do not use it.

Some of the exercises are performed on the floor (please use a mat or carpeted area if possible) so, the only equipment you will be using will be your own body weight, and you can take that anywhere.

It's Not Too Late!

PROGRESSION

Part of our modern American culture is the idea that "more is better". This mentality is possibly responsible for more exercise injuries than you could imagine. When an individual starts an exercise program, there are many different theories out there. In fact there are so many, how can they help **not** being confused? One "guru" says this and another says that, and on and on until the individual is so confused that they will often, especially in a health club environment, seeks out the person who looks the best.

Big mistake! That good looking well muscled person looks that way for many reasons. One reason is genetics. They have also probably been exercising for a long time. Here is where a lot of problems start. If that person does five to six sets of each exercise and it works for them they most likely will tell you that you should do the same. If you are just starting out, you cannot **possibly** perform up to the standards of a long time fitness buff—especially one who is—ahem—much younger.

Proper progression is possibly the most important piece to the fitness puzzle. Not using proper progression is what will get you in trouble. It seems that new exercisers continuously will push themselves to the limit from the very start, usually trying to lift too much weight or do too many reps.

It's Not Too Late! teaches a different approach to fitness; one that encompasses proper form, proper progression, patience and common sense. The concept of "no pain no gain" is old and silly. If you feel you are straining, then you are! It's that simple. If you can do ten reps of an exercise on Monday and can still only do ten reps on Wednesday that **is** okay! Rome was not built in a day and neither will your new body.

In the beginners program, we will be working in the 8 to 12 range of repetitions. We will have you start out with 8 repetitions on each exercise, slowly working your way to 12. Not everyone will be able to perform 8 repetitions at first. Then if that is the case, use 5 to 8 repetitions as your starting point. If you can't perform 5, just do as many as you can. There is no competition here, and this is certainly not a race. As we stated before you should **always check with your physician(s) before beginning an exercise program.**

Okay! Now, you have established your starting point. As you perform each exercise you must strive to add an additional rep or two, as you feel your body can handle it, until you can perform at the top of your range. If you are performing 8 reps in the beginning keep working until you can reach

12. Your muscle groups will adapt, little by little, until you reach your goals. Remember; never try to blast a muscle into growth— gentle coaxing works so much better. It's time to get started. So, here we go!

Beginning Workout Instruction

This section assumes that you are a beginner and new to physical culture. There are some important things to know before you begin using this exercise system or any other.

CAUTION: Anyone starting an exercise program for the first time should always check with their physician to see if they may have any problems that could be exacerbated by exercise. Second, a physician can also outline any contraindications to exercise that would reduce the risk of worsening an existing condition.

Keep in mind that to achieve any reward such as improved fitness there are always risks. There is the risk of after-work out soreness or even injury. We have been very careful in preparing our programs at all levels to avoid this from happening, but we just want you to be prepared that these things can possibly happen.

POSTURE

When we were kids we always got sick of hearing our mother tell us to stand up straight. Well, I guess you can start calling me 'Mom' because that's just what I am going to do. I am going to teach you how to stand up straight. View the photo below:

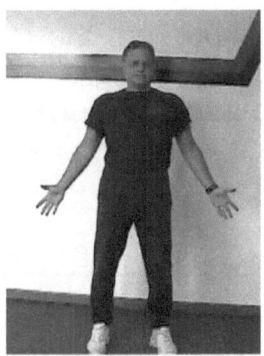

As you can see I am standing in the anatomical position with shoulders pulled back and down. The rib cage is depressed to tighten the abdominals. The glutes (butt) are pulled tight. I call this the **altogether position**. While in this position, you are stable and less prone to injure yourself. See side view of this position below:

It's Not Too Late!

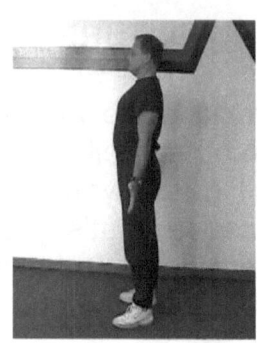

While you perform the movements in this book I want you to try and maintain this **altogether position** whenever possible, especially during the exercises where you are standing.

USING THE EXERCISE SHEETS

There are fifteen different exercises in the Beginning Workout. Each exercise has an instruction sheet with photos designed to help you perform them properly and safely. You will also see that the sheets provide additional information, such as the purpose for performing the exercise, as well listing what muscles are being used in the action. This will help you understand what changes you will be attempting to make in your body. **Remember, if you feel any pain or feel any discomfort other than your muscles and joints working, stop immediately and call your physician**.

HOW TO EXERCISE

We recommend that you warm up a bit before you start your exercise session. If you have a treadmill or an exercise bike, 5-10 minutes at a slow to moderate pace should be enough. If you do not have this type of equipment, a short walk outside or walking in place will do. **Do not get out of breath!** If you do you are probably exercising at too quick a pace. Remember, all we are doing during the warm-up is getting the joints moving and elevate your core body temperature.

Once you have properly warmed up, proceed with the first exercise listed. All the exercises should be performed slow and strict (as shown in the photos). A cadence of 1,2,3,4 count up and 1,2,3,4 count down works very well. As we have already stated, this is not a race or a contest. If you cannot do the exercise in this cadence, please modify it to your comfort level until you can. It is very important to perform the exercises in the order given. Doing so eliminates the need for stretching after your session. **If, after the workout, you feel the need to stretch, please contact a fitness professional to learn the proper form. Stretching can cause injuries if performed improperly.**

It's Not Too Late!

You should try to perform the Beginning Workout a minimum of twice a week for five weeks or until you feel that you are ready to add one more session per week. At this time, we recommend one, two or three exercise sessions per week or every other day. Work at your own pace—whatever you can handle. We **do not** recommend everyday or two days in a row.

Start with one set at the 8-12 rep range if possible. Use the lightest resistance at first, working up slowly to the next level Remember, if you cannot perform 8 reps try 5 or 3 and work your way up to 8. Once you can do 8 reps, then work your way up to 12. After you have reached 12 reps in an exercise then add a second set and do as many as you can until you can perform 12 reps in the second set as well. Once you can perform three sets of 12 of each exercise you will then be ready for the Intermediate Workout.

If you have any questions on how to perform any exercises or how to use the equipment provided you can e-mail your questions to us at **tfcon@comcast.net.** We will answer your questions free of charge for two weeks after the first inquiry. After the first two weeks we will offer a yearly subscription for technical support through our website.

It's Not Too Late!

For more information, please e-mail the above address.

HIP EXTENSION

The Hip Extension strengthens the hip extensors and hamstrings.

When performing this movement you will be turning on (working) the Gluteus Maximus and hamstring muscles while turning off (relaxing) the hip flexors and quadriceps.

Lie face down on floor or flat bench, placing hands beneath your hips. Raise one leg towards the ceiling from the hip without losing contact with your hands, pause and return to start position. **Special instructions:** To increase resistance place band, around ankles.

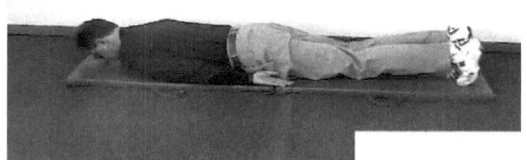

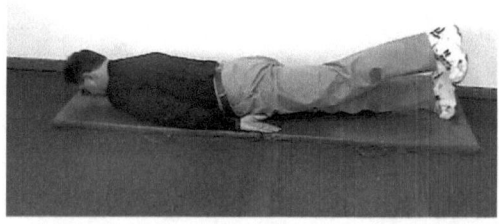

REVERSE TORSO CURL

The Reverse Torso Curl will strengthen the lower abdominal muscles while relaxing the lower back muscles. Proper development of the abdominal muscles is important for low back stability and maintaining good posture.
When performing this movement you will be firing (working) lower abdominals, Internal and external oblique and Transverse Abdominus. To perform the reverse torso, lie on back on flat surface or bench. Bring knees up toward chest until knees are over belt line. Contract the lower abdominals and curl pelvic area up to approximately 2 inches off the surface, keeping the mid-back in contact with the surface. Hold, and then return to start position.

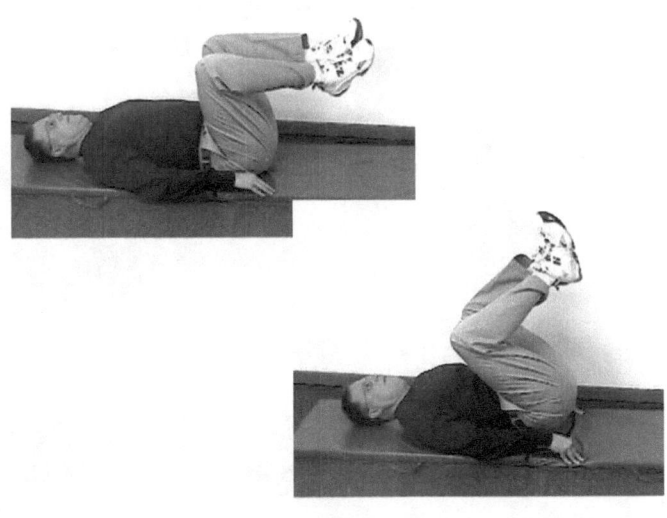

SCAPULAR PROTRACTIONS

The Scapular Protraction exercise strengthens the Serratus Anterior muscle. The serratus muscle is a stabilizer for the scapular (shoulder blade) during upper body movements. Performing this movement will fire (work) Serratus Anterior and the Pectoralis Major, while relaxing the Rhomboids.

When performing this movement, attach the tubing at approximately shoulder height. Stand with your back to the tubing. While holding the tubing handle in your right hand straighten your arm out in front of your body at shoulder level and step forward to remove any slack in tube or cable. With elbow straight, push tubing away from your body by rounding your shoulders, pause and return to start position. **Do not turn your body during the exercise—this will keep the targeted muscles from doing the work.**

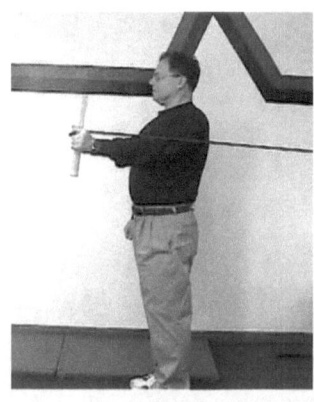 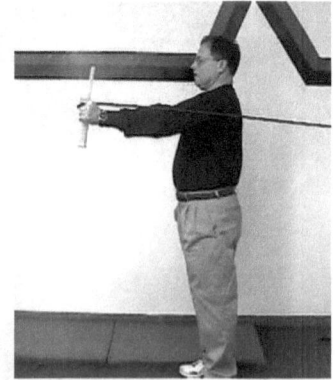

SEATED ROW

The seated row exercise will strengthen the mid back and posterior shoulder muscles. This movement works the Latissimus Dorsi, Posterior Deltoid and Rhomboid muscles.

When performing this movement, Sit facing the weight stack and hold each handle. Back up to remove slack in the tube. Pull your shoulders back and down. Pull your elbows back until they are next to your body. Hold and slowly return to the starting position.

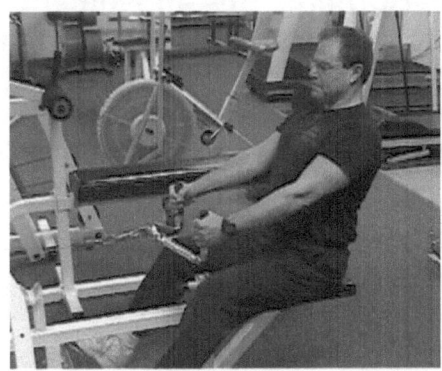

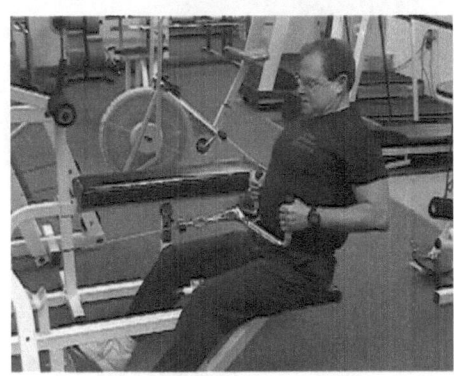

SHOULDER ADDUCTION ON A DIAGONAL PLANE

Shoulder adduction on a diagonal plane strengthens the anterior shoulder and chest muscles. It is an excellent PNF (proprioceptive neuromuscular facilitation) exercise for the pectorals (chest muscles) and to reset the posterior shoulder muscles. On this movement, you will work the Pectoralis Major, Anterior Deltoid muscles.

When performing this movement, secure end of tubing overhead, hold handle with arm extended to side overhead with palm facing forward. Pull handle across body until palm is facing hip. Hold and return to starting position. Turn around and repeat other side.

Exercise can be performed on pulley equipment as well using same directions.

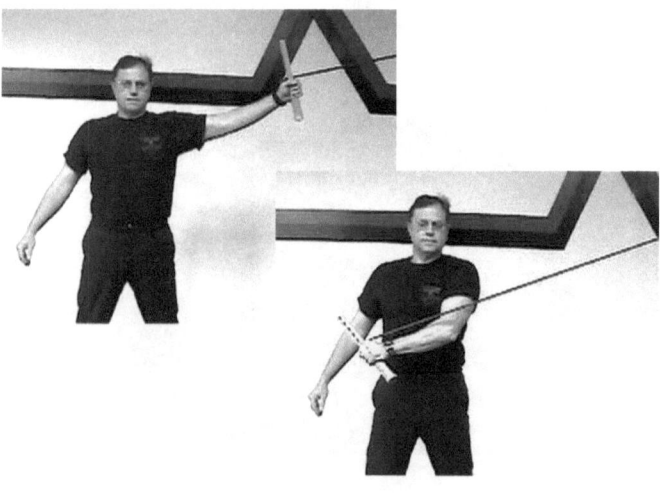

SEATED KNEE EXTENSIONS

Seated knee extensions are a great exercise to strengthen the quadriceps muscles, reset the hamstrings and stabilize the knee joint. Performing this movement works the Vastus Medialis, Lateralis, Intermedius and Rectus Femoris muscles, while relaxing the hamstrings.

When performing this movement, sit on machine with lower legs hanging over the bench behind ankle pads. Keep shoulders back and sit up straight maintaining a straight back. Slowly extend lower legs until straight. Hold and slowly return to the starting position.

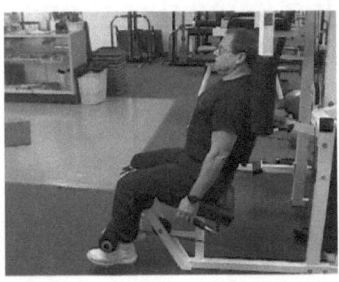

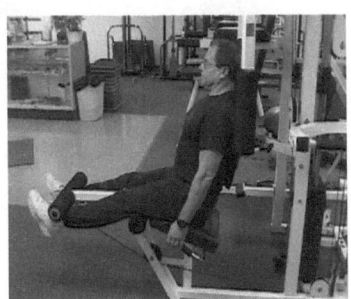

SHOULDER EXTENSION

Shoulder Extensions will improve posture while strengthening the posterior shoulder, back and triceps. To perform this movement you will be firing the Latissimus Dorsi, Teres Major, triceps and Posterior Deltoids. Secure tube at top of door or other immovable object.

When performing this movement, face whatever the tube is attached to, hold an end of the tube in one hand. With elbow slightly bent, start with arm at chest level. Squeeze your shoulder blades back and down. With arms straight, pull tubing down past your hip, pause and return to starting position.

Exercise can be performed on pulley equipment as well using same directions.

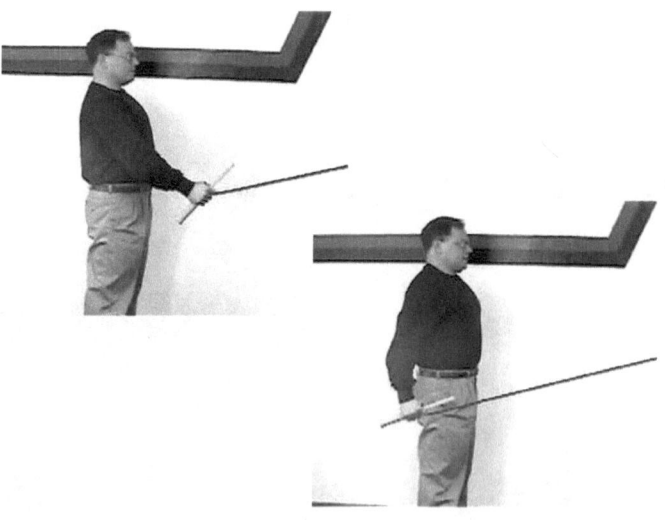

SHOULDER HORIZONTAL ABDUCTION

The Shoulder Abduction exercise will strengthen the posterior shoulder muscles while relaxing the chest and anterior shoulder muscles. Performing this movement will turn on the Posterior Deltoid and Rhomboids muscles while turning off the Pectorals.

When performing this movement secure tubing at shoulder level. Stand with right side facing the secured strap. Hold handle in left hand and hold directly in front at about chest level. With elbow slightly bent, pull tubing away from secured end until arm is straight out to side. Turn to other side and repeat directions. Reps are to be performed in a slow, controlled manner.

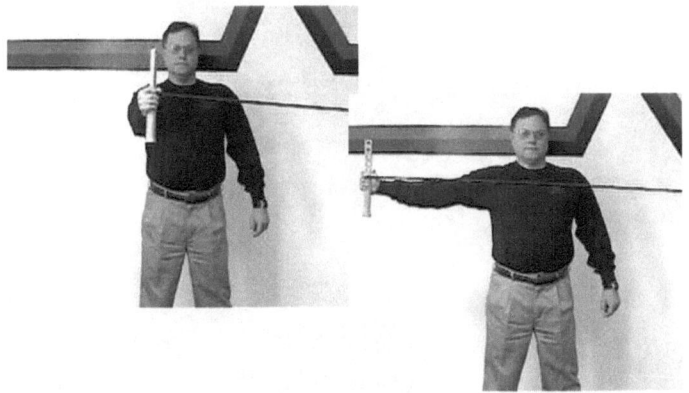

Exercise can be performed on pulley equipment as well using same directions.

BRIDGES

Bridges are great for strengthening the core. It works the lower abs, glutes, and spinal erectors and improves spinal stability. This movement works the Erector Spinae, Gluteus Maximus, Hamstrings, Lower Abdominals, and the oblique muscles.
When performing this movement, lie face up on flat surface; keep both legs bent with feet on floor at shoulder width. Contract your abdominals and slowly lift your hips towards the ceiling until you feel your glutes lock up forcing you to stop. Keep your core in line by leading with your pelvic area. Hold and lower back to the starting position

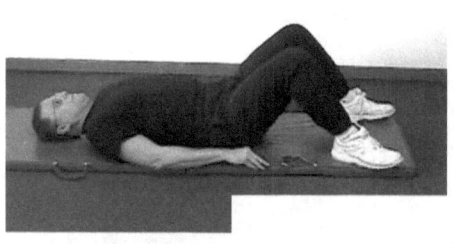

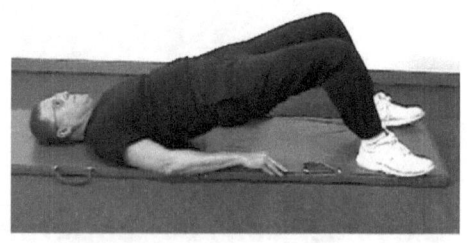

ABDOMINAL CURL (CRUNCH)

The Abdominal Crunch strengthens the upper abdominal muscles. The abdominals are important in maintaining posture and providing back stability. The abdominal muscles when contracted will relax the middle and upper back muscles. This movement works the Rectus Abdominus, Internal and External Obliques and Transverse Abdominus.

When performing this movement, lie on your back on the floor. Place feet up on bench or chair and pull your knees back so they are over your belt line. Tuck your chin (press back of neck down to surface) and gently press your heels down against the bench or chair. Slowly curl your upper torso, bringing your shoulders towards your knees keeping your chin tucked and the lower back in contact with the surface. Hold and slowly lower until shoulders contact surface. Repeat.

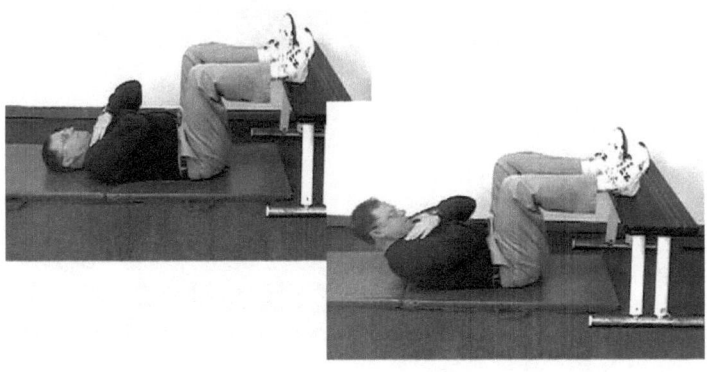

HIP FLEXION

The Hip Flexion exercise will strengthen the powerful hip flexors while relaxing the hip extensors. **Do not perform this exercise if you are experiencing lower back pain.** This movement will fire up the Iliopsoas, Sartorius and Rectus Femoris muscles while relaxing the hamstrings and glutes.

When performing this movement, lie on the floor on your back. Maintain a flat lower back throughout the movement. Lift leg straight up until you cannot go any higher without the leg flexing at the knee. Do not bring it up higher than 90 degrees, hold at the top of the movement, then slowly lower leg to start position, repeat with other leg.

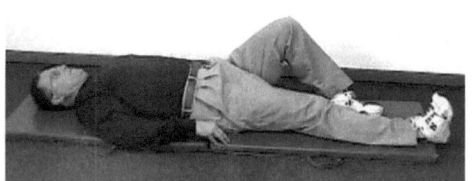

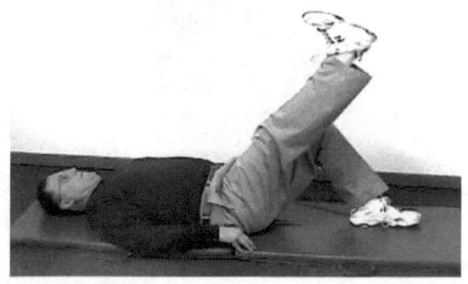

SHOULDER HYPERFLEXION

The Shoulder Hyperflexion strengthens the upper back muscles and improves posture. As these muscles act as stabilizers for the shoulder joint, proper development can help prevent injury. When performing this movement, you will be firing (working) the Middle and Lower Trapezius, Posterior Deltoids and Rhomboids.

When performing this movement attach tubing to about waist height. Face the anchor and grab the handle with both hands facing down. With your arms straight and out in front of your body with your shoulders pulled back and down, slowly raise your arms up until the handle is overhead. Pause at the top and return to start position. **Do not lean backwards while performing this exercise.**

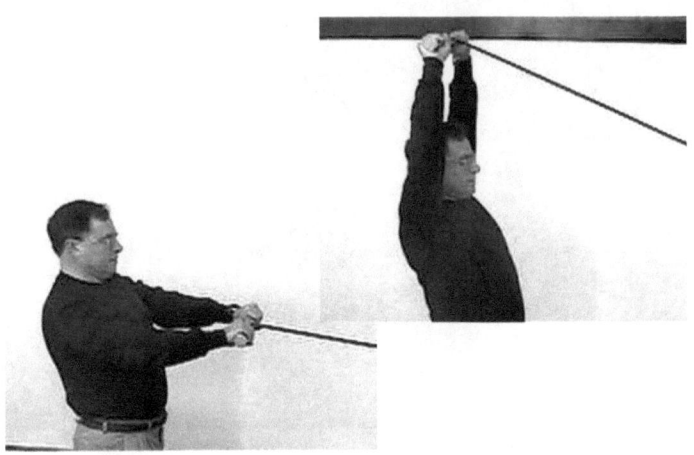

LATERAL TORSO BRIDGE

The Lateral Torso Bridge exercise strengthens the trunk lateral flexor muscles. This movement works the Internal & External Obliques, Transverse Abdominus and Quadratus Lumborum

When performing this movement, lie on the floor or flat bench on your side. Bend at the side and prop the upper body up on the elbow. Slowly raise the lower torso until body is straight. Pause and lower to start position.

Special Instructions: If exercise is too difficult, bend knees to 90 degrees.

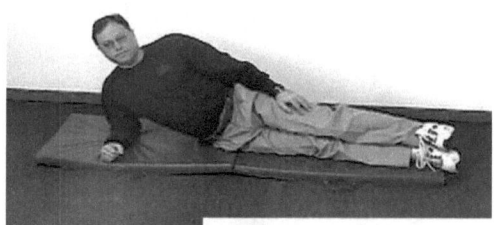

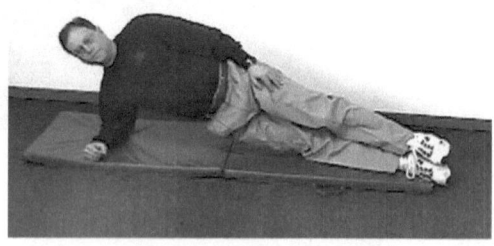

INTERMEDIATE WORKOUT

This section assumes that you have completed the Beginning Workout sections of this book and that you feel ready to progress to the Intermediate level. If you attempt to work at this level and find it too difficult, please return to the Beginning phase of this training until you are ready to progress.

There are some important things to know before you begin using this exercise system or any other exercise program.

CAUTION: Anyone starting an exercise program for the first time should always check with their physician to see if they may have any problems that could be made worse with exercise. Second, a physician can also outline any contraindications to exercise that would reduce the risk of making a condition worse. If that is the case we can make adjustments in the existing program to compensate at no extra charge so you can exercise safely.

CAUTION: It is very important that the equipment that you use whether it is at your gym or in your home be well maintained and in good working order. If there is any doubt that this is the case, do not use it.

It's Not Too Late!

USING THE EXERCISE SHEETS

There are fifteen different exercises in the Intermediate Workout. Each exercise has an instruction sheet with photos designed to help you perform them properly and safely. You will also see that the sheets provide additional information such as the purpose for performing the exercise as well as telling you what muscles are being used in the action. This will help you understand what changes you will be making in your body. Remember if you feel any pain or discomfort or feel anything other than your muscles and joints working, stop immediately and contact your physician.

HOW TO EXERCISE

We recommend that you warm up a bit before you start your exercise session. If you have a treadmill or an exercise bike, 5-10 minutes at a slow to moderate pace should be enough. If you do not have this type of equipment a short walk outside or walking in place will do. **Do not get out of breath!** If you do, you are probably exercising at too fast of a pace. Remember all we are doing is getting the body to move and elevate your core temperature. Another very effective warm up is to perform one set of the Beginning Workout before your Intermediate Workout. This should be adequate to warm up those joints and muscles.

PROGRESSION

In the Intermediate program we will be working in the 8 to 12 range of repetitions. We will have you start out with 8 repetitions on each exercise slowly working your way to 12. Start with the green tube and the red band as the lightest resistance, working your way up to the blue tube as the heaviest resistance. When performing the exercises on pulley equipment start with a resistance that you can do 12 repetitions. If you experience difficulty in performing in this rep range then you are not ready to progress and we recommend that you continue using the Beginning Workout for another week or two before returning to the Intermediate Workout again. There is no competition here and this is certainly not a race. Also, as we stated before you should always check with your physician before, beginning an exercise program.

Okay! Now you have established your Intermediate starting point. Now as you perform each exercise you must strive to add an additional rep or two, as you feel your

It's Not Too Late!

body can handle it, until you can perform at the top of your range. If you can perform 8 repetitions, keep working until you can reach 12. Your muscle groups will adapt, little by little, until you reach your goals. Remember, never try to blast a muscle into growth; gentle coaxing works much better.

SHOULDER FLEXION

The Shoulder Flexion exercise will strengthen the anterior shoulder muscles.

Performing this exercise will work the Anterior Deltoid muscle with the Biceps and Coracobrachialis muscles assisting the movement.

When performing this movement, anchor the tubing at floor level (stepping on tube as shown). Start with your arm down to your side. Grip the handle of the tube. Lock elbow and wrist and raise the handle straight out in front of you until it is at shoulder height. Pause then return slowly to the start position.

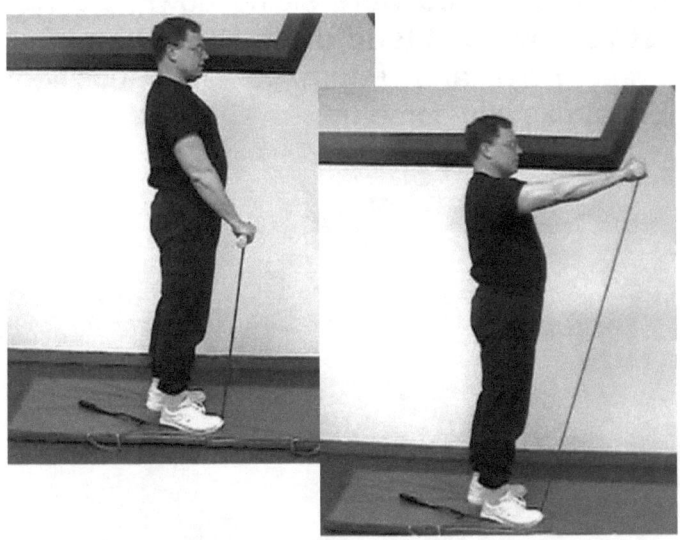

Exercise can be performed with pulley or free weights as well using same direction

STATIONARY LUNGE

The Stationary Lunge exercise is a lower body closed chain exercise that will strengthen the abductors and hip flexion muscles.

When performing this movement, you will be working the Gluteus Mudius and Minimus the Rectus Femoris, Tensor Fascia Lata and the Psoas muscles.

Stand with one foot out in front and the other slightly back. (See top photo) Carefully position the front foot so the knee lines up with your big toe. While keeping your weight on the heel of the front foot, drop down from the hip as if you were sitting down. **Do not let your knee extend out further than your toes.** Hold and return to start position. Exhale as you come up.

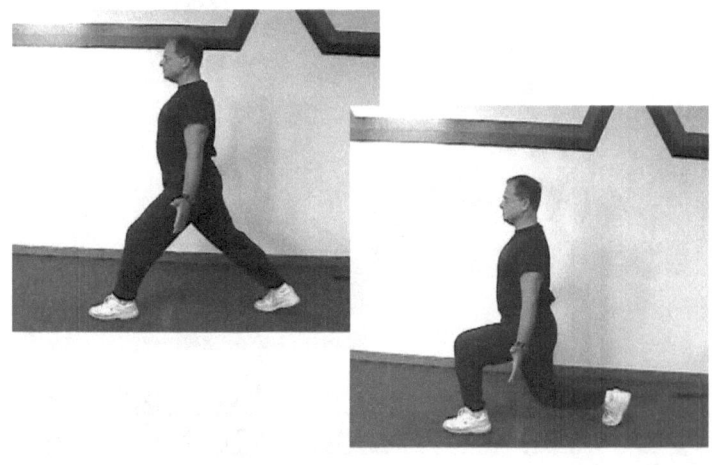

SHOULDER ABDUCTION ON A DIAGONAL PLANE

The Shoulder Abduction on a Diagonal Plane exercise will strengthen the posterior shoulder muscles while relaxing the chest and anterior shoulder muscles. This PNF movement will improve posture and shoulder stability. This movement works the Posterior Deltoid, Rhomboids, Mid and Lower Trapezius, while relaxing the Pectoralis muscles.

When performing this movement, secure tubing at floor level. Stand with right side facing the secured tubing. Hold handle in left hand.

With left hand at hip level, palm facing your body and elbow slightly bent. Bring your arm up and out until it is over your left shoulder. Hold and return to starting position. Repeat. Turn to other side and repeat directions. Reps are to be performed in a slow, controlled manner.

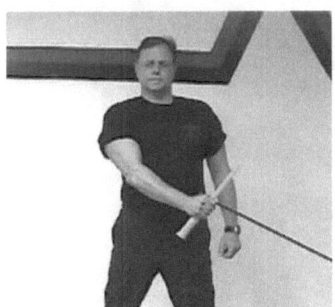 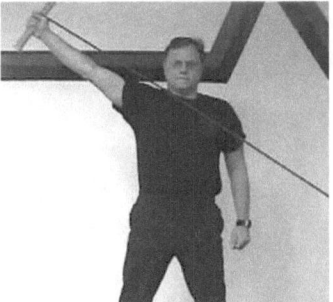

SPINAL EXTENSION

The Spinal Extension exercise strengthens the low back muscles. This is an excellent exercise for improving posture. Erector Spinae and the Latissimus Dorsi are the muscles the muscles turning on while the abdominal muscles relax.

When performing this movement, lie face down on flat surface. The floor or a flat bench will work. Tuck your chin so you are looking straight down at the floor. Pinch the shoulder blades (Scapula retraction) together, exhale and slowly raise your chest off the floor. As you come up, rotate your shoulders so your thumbs are pointing towards the ceiling. Hold and slowly lower yourself to the starting position.

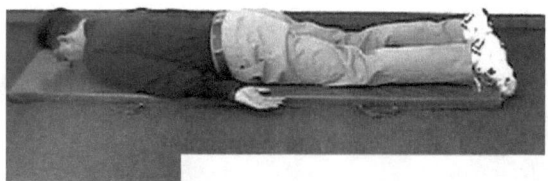

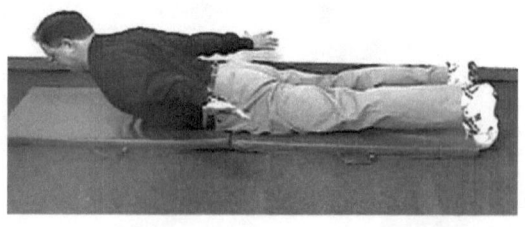

SHOULDER ABDUCTION

Shoulder Abduction with tubing is a great exercise to strengthen the Deltoid Muscles, the Anterior, Lateral and Posterior Deltoids. Stand on end of tubing. Stand with your side facing where the tubing is attached.

When performing this movement, take tubing handle in your hand with palm facing your body. Lock your elbow and slowly raise your arm until it is at shoulder level. Pause, and then return to the starting position.

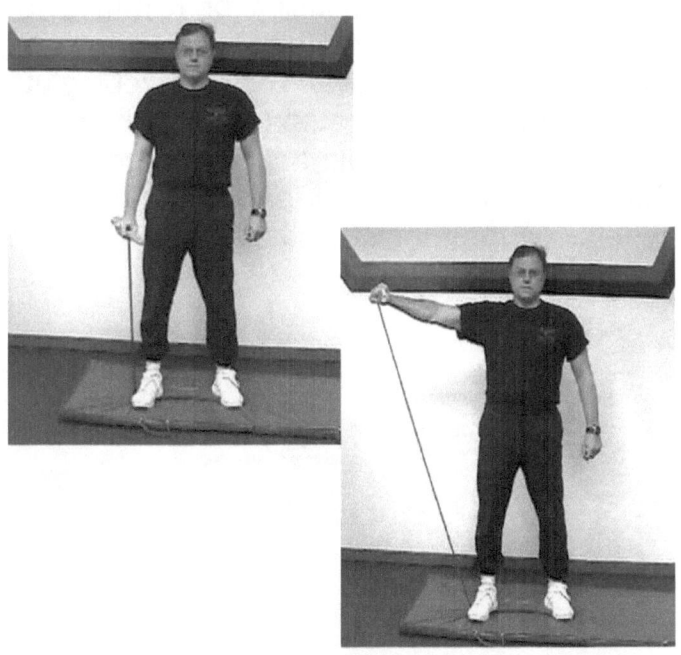

Exercise can be performed with pulley or free weights as well using same direction

LOW SPINAL EXTENSION

The Low Spinal Extension exercise will strengthen the muscles of the low back and hips. (This is an advanced exercise for the lower back and should not be attempted until you are ready).Performing this movement works the Erector Spinae, Latissimus Dorsi, Quadratus Lumborum, Gluteus Maximus and Hamstrings

When performing this movement, lie face down on flat surface, preferably a bench, hold on to the bench using both hands for support. Keep leg straight and slowly lift towards the ceiling until you feel your glute lock up forcing you to stop (or as high as you can without pain). Hold and lower leg to the starting position. Perform specified repetitions then repeat with other leg.

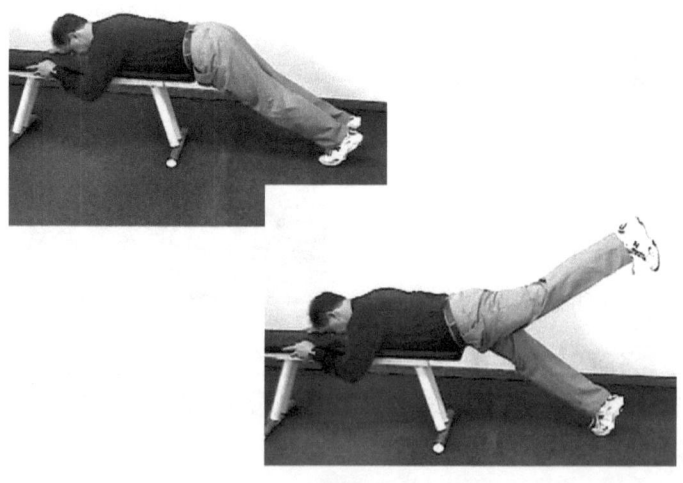

ABDOMINAL CRUNCH WITH ROTATION

The Abdominal Crunch with Rotation strengthens the abdominal muscles and relaxes the muscles of the middle and upper back.

The muscles worked are the Rectus Abdominus and the Obliques, internal and external.

When performing this movement, lie on a flat surface with your feet up on a chair or bench. Make sure that your knees are directly over your belt line. Tuck your chin (press your neck down toward the flat surface) and press your heels gently into the bench. Slowly curl upper body up off the surface. While in this position, twist your torso so that your left shoulder is reaching for your right knee. Return to the centered position and then slowly return to the start position.

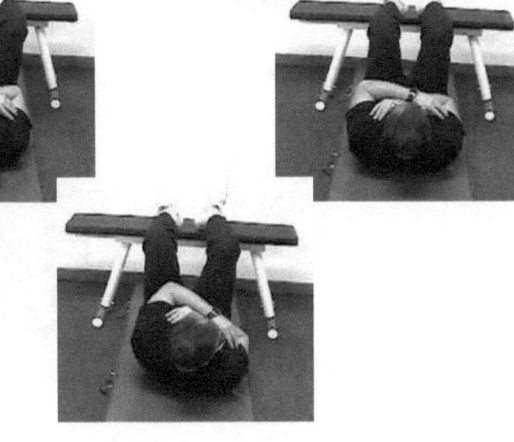

SHOULDER ADDUCTION - LAT PULL DOWN

The Shoulder Adduction exercise will strengthen the Latissimus Dorsi, Teres Major and Pectoral Major muscle groups while relaxing the shoulder abductors.

When performing this movement Grasp lat bar with hands placed just beyond shoulder width. Keeping arms straight, pull your shoulders back and down. Once set pull bar to just below chin. Hold and slowly return to the start position.

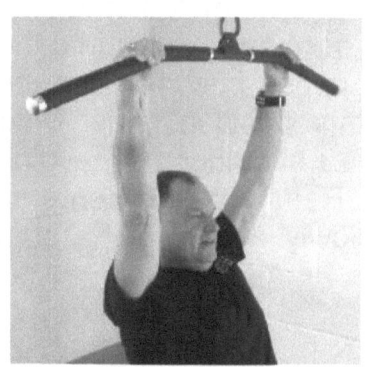

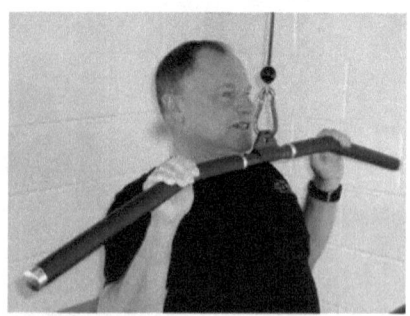

ROW WITH TUBING

The Row with Tubing exercise will strengthen the mid back and posterior shoulder muscles. This movement works the Latissimus Dorsi, Posterior Deltoid and Rhomboids muscles.

When performing this movement, attach the tubing at (wrap around pole or other immovable vertical object) chest level. Stand facing the anchor and hold each handle. Back up to remove slack in the tube. Pull your shoulders back and down. Pull your elbows back until they are next to your body. Hold and slowly return to the starting position.

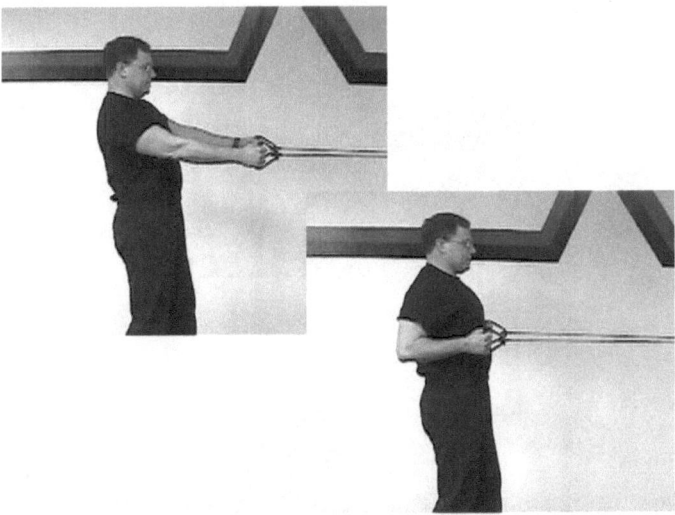

Exercise can be performed with pulley machine as well using same directions.

LATERAL TORSO BRIDGE

The Lateral Torso Bridge exercise strengthens the trunk lateral flexor muscles. Performing this movement works the Internal & External Obliques, Transverse Abdominus and Quadratus Lumborum.

When performing this movement, lie on the floor or flat bench on your side. Bend at the side and prop the upper body up on the elbow. Slowly raise the lower torso until body is straight. Pause and lower to start position.

Special Instructions: If exercise is too difficult, bend knees to 90 degrees.

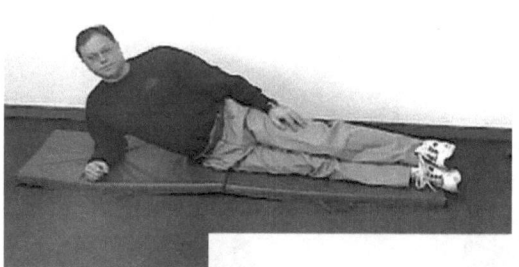

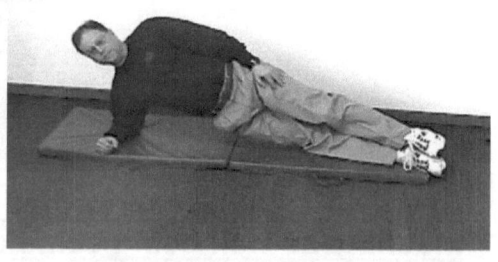

LEG PRESS

The leg press is great for strengthening the Gluteus Maximus, Hamstrings, and Quadriceps.

When performing this movement, lie or sit in machine and place feet on deck at about shoulder with. With toes pointing slightly away from each other, press on deck emphasizing the heels until legs straighten. Do no lock knees! Stop just short of lock-out and return to start position. If you are on a machine with a weight stack do not allow weights to touch.

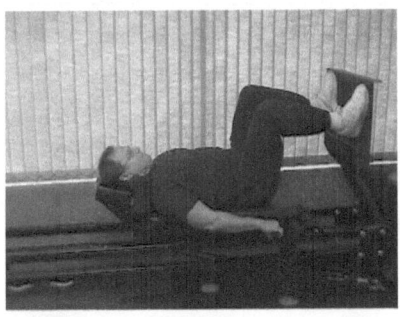

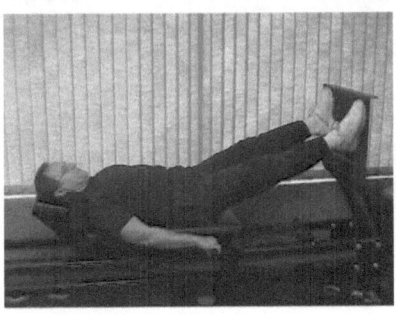

REVERSE TORSO CURL WITH LATERAL FLEXION

The Reverse Torso Curl with Lateral Flexion will strengthen the lower abdominal and Oblique muscles while relaxing the lower back muscles. Proper development of the abdominal muscles is important for lower back stability and maintaining good posture. You will be firing (working) the Lower Abdominals, Internal and External Obliques and Transversus Abdominus.

When performing this movement, lie on back on flat surface or bench. Bring knees up toward chest until knees are over belt line. Contract the lower abdominals and curl pelvic area up to about 2 inches off the surface. Keeping the back in contact with the surface, crunch the right hip toward shoulder, return to start position, repeat, crunching left hip to left shoulder.

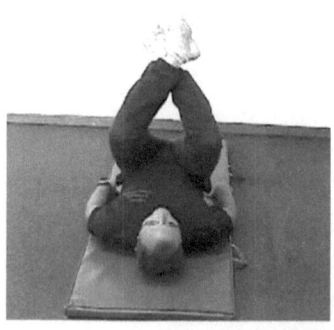 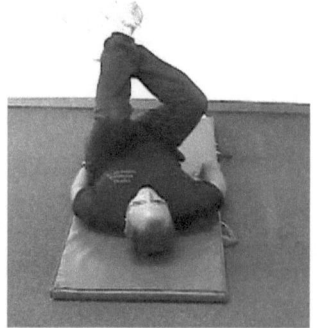

It's Not Too Late!

Advanced Workout

This section assumes that you have completed the Beginning and Intermediate Workout sections and that you feel ready to progress to the Advanced level.

There are some important things to know before you begin using this exercise system or any other exercise program.

CAUTION: First, anyone starting an exercise program for the first time should always check with their physician to see if they may have any problems that could be made worse with exercise. Second, a physician can also outline any contraindications to exercise that would reduce the risk of making a condition worse. If that is the case, we suggest contacting a qualified fitness trainer in your area to assist you in making these adjustments to the program.

Keep in mind that to achieve any reward such as improved fitness there is always a risk. There is a risk of after work out soreness or even injury. We have been very careful in preparing our programs at all levels to hopefully avoid this from happening, but we just want

you to be prepared that these things can possibly happen.

USING THE EXERCISE SHEETS

There are thirteen different exercises in the Advanced Workout. Each exercise has an instruction sheet with photos designed to help you perform them properly and safely. You will also see that the sheets provide additional information such as the purpose for performing the exercise as well as describing what muscles are being used in the action. This will help you understand what changes you will be making to your body. **Remember if you feel any pain or feel any discomfort other than your muscles and joints working stop immediately and contact your physician**.

HOW TO EXERCISE

We recommend that you warm up a bit before you start your exercise session. If you have treadmill or an exercise bike, 5-10 minutes at a slow to moderate pace should be enough. If you do not have this type of equipment, a short walk outside or walking in place will do. **Do not get out of breath!** If you do you are probably exercising at too fast a pace. Remember, all we are doing is getting the body to move and elevate your core temperature. Another very effective warm up is to perform one set of the Beginning Workout before your Advanced Workout. This should be adequate to warm up those joints and muscles.

In this section, on certain exercises, you will be adding **Terminal Flicks.** These flicks are to be performed at the end of a set. At the last repetition we will end at the terminal point (the top or extreme end of the movement) hold, then quickly flick between the top of the movement and the last ten degrees. Start with five flicks and work your way to twenty. This additional movement will build strength and stamina.

All the exercises should be performed slow and strict (as shown in the photos). A cadence of 1,2,3,4 count up and 1,2,3,4 count down works very well. As we stated before this is not a race or a contest. **If you cannot do the exercise in this cadence please modify it to your comfort level until you can.** It is very important to perform the exercises in the order given. Doing so eliminates the need for stretching after your session.

It's Not Too Late!

You should try to perform the Advanced Workout a minimum of twice a week. We recommend three times per week. We do not recommend performing the exercises everyday or two days in a row.

We recommend that you start in the one set, 8-12 rep range if possible. Remember, if you cannot perform 8 reps at this level go back to the Intermediate Workout until you are able to do 8 reps. Once you can do 8 reps work your way up to 12. After you have reached 12 reps in an exercise then add a second set and do as many as you can until you can perform 12 reps in the second set as well. Once you can perform three sets of 12 of each exercise you will then be ready for a split routine that is outlined below. Here's where you get to use all the tubing and bands, depending of course on your individual strength level, on some exercises you should be able to use the purple tube. When performing these split routines, we have added exercises from the Beginning and Intermediate Workouts.

EXTERNAL SHOULDER ROTATION

The External Shoulder Rotation is a great movement for improved posture and is great for shoulder strength. External rotation of the shoulder in the closed pack position will also strengthen the muscles of the rotator cuff as it relaxes the pectorals and the anterior shoulder muscles. Muscles used are the Supraspranitus, Infraspinitus and Teres Minor.

When performing this movement, secure tubing at about shoulder level. Facing the tubing, hold handle in one hand with your palm facing the floor. With the elbow bent at 90 degrees at shoulder level and your upper arm parallel to the floor, rotate your shoulder bringing your hand toward the ceiling. Hold and return to start position.

SPECIAL INSTRUCTIONS: It is very important to keep your upper arm parallel to floor. Add Terminal Flicks when ready.

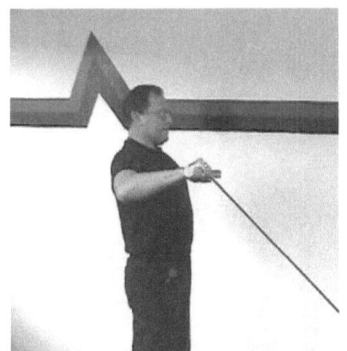 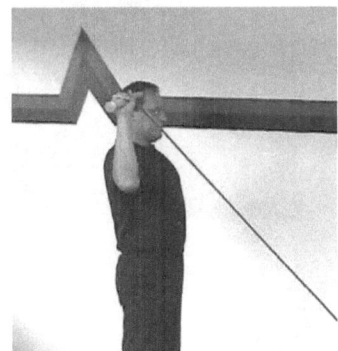

SINGLE LEG CALF RAISE

The standing single leg calf raise exercise will develop the Gastrocnemius and the Soleus muscles of the calves.

When performing this movement, stand on a block to elevate the foot. Place one foot behind the heel of the other. With the ball of the foot on the block let the heel drop below the level of the block. **Do not drop your heel any further than just below the block. Full stretch of the Achilles tendon under the load of your body weight can cause injury.** Push your body up by flexing your ankle until you cannot go any higher. Hold and then return to start position.

SPECIAL INSTRUCTIONS: Add Terminal Flicks at the end of the set when ready.

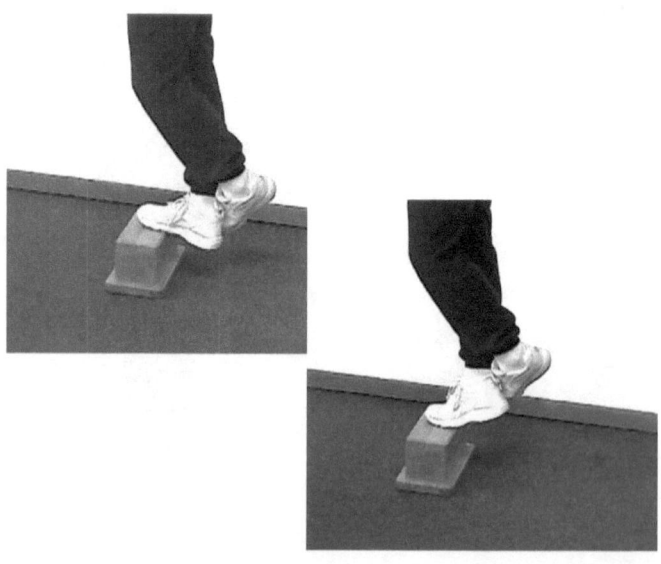

SQUATS

The Squat is a great full body workout that emphasizes the upper leg and gluteal area. This movement works the Quadaceps, and Gluteal muscles.

When performing this movement, stand up straight up and down with the tubing under your feet (at shoulder width toes pointing out slightly). Holding a handle in each hand flex knees until upper leg is at approximately a 45-degree angle. **Knees should not go forward beyond the toes for proper knee tracking.** Hold and then return to start position.

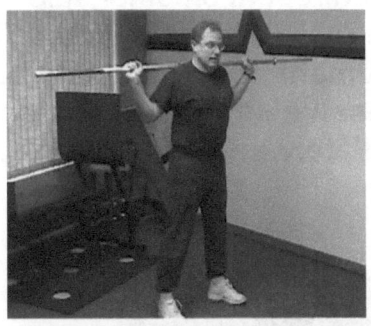

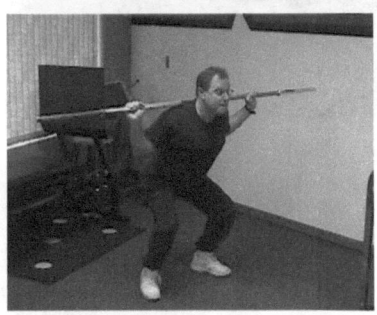

LATERAL BRIDGE WITH ROTATION

The Lateral Torso Bridge with Rotation exercise strengthens the trunk lateral flexor and rotation muscles. Performing this movement works the Internal & External Obliques, Transverse Abdominus and Quadratus Lumborum

When performing this movement, lie on the floor or flat bench on your side. Bend at the side and prop the upper body up on the elbow. Slowly raise the lower torso until body is straight. While holding this position, turn your upper torso toward the floor. After you complete the repetitions, lower to start position and repeat on other side.

CAUTION: This is a very difficult movement. If you feel any pain or excessive strain, stop exercising immediately and call your physician.

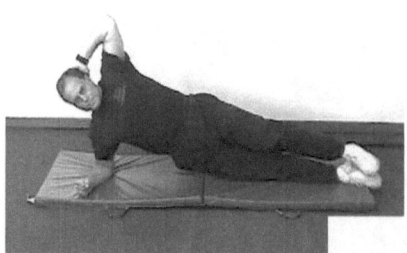

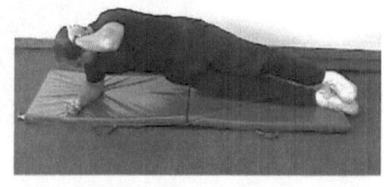

STEP AND PRESS

The Step and Press is a full body workout that will emphasize the Pectoralis Major, Anterior Deltoid, Quadraceps and the Abdominal Muscles. This movement is excellent for core stability and for strengthening the upper body.

When performing this movement, wrap the tubing around a fixed object at shoulder height with your back facing it. Holding your arms at your sides at shoulder level, step out to a lunge position. At the same time push your arms out in front at a slight downward angle, then return to start position.

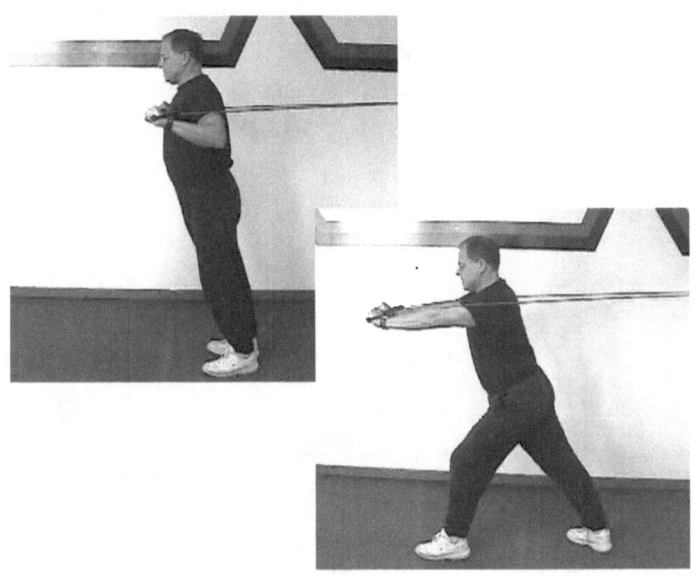

<u>LOW SPINAL EXTENSION</u>

The Low Spinal Extension exercise will strengthen the muscles of the lower back and hips. (This is an advanced exercise for the lower back and should not be attempted until you are ready).This movement works the Erector Spinae, Latissimus Dorsi, Quadratus Lumborum, Gluteus Maximus and Hamstrings while relaxing the hip flexors.

Lie face down on flat surface, preferably a bench; hold on to the bench using both hands for support. Keep both legs straight and slowly lift towards the ceiling until you feel your glutes lock up forcing you to stop or as high as you can without pain. Hold and lower legs to the starting position.

CAUTION: This is a very difficult movement. If you feel any pain or excessive strain, stop exercising immediately and call your physician.

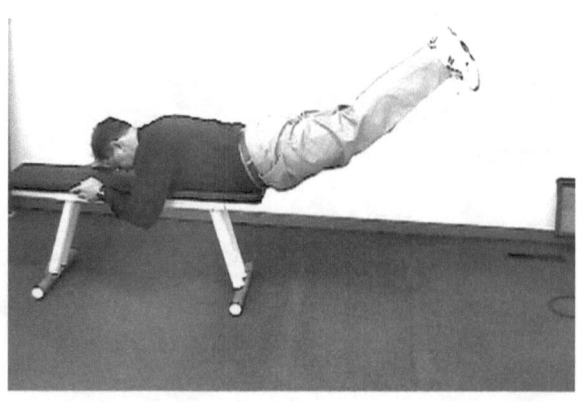

BENCH PRESS

The Bench Press is a full body workout that will emphasize the Pectoralis Major, Anterior Deltoid.

When performing this movement, place hands on bar just outside shoulder with, lift bar from rack until elbows are straight. Move bar over chest, squeeze shoulder blades together then lower bar until upper arm is parallel to floor. (Bar does not need to touch chest). Slowly push up bar until elbows are straight but short of lock-out.

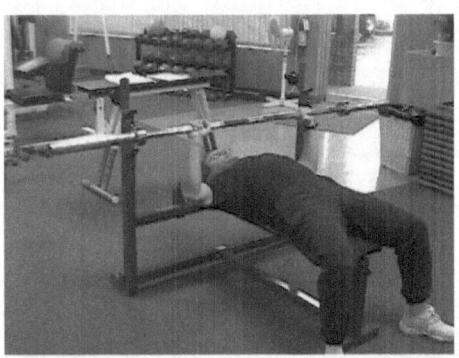

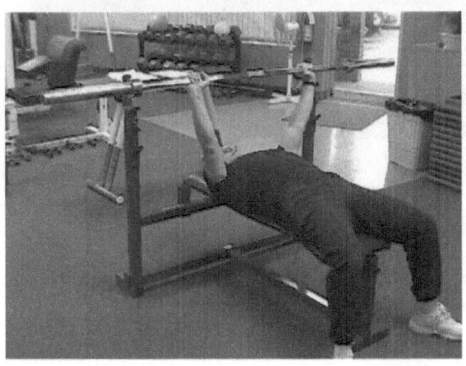

SINGLE ARM ROW

The Single Arm Row is a great upper body strengthening exercise. This exercise will help achieve balance with the usually tight Pectoral muscles. This movement works the Rhomboids, Latissimus Dorsi and rear Deltoids
muscles.
When performing this movement, attach tubing at floor level. Stand facing the tubing. Hold both ends in one hand. Open up stance by placing one foot in front of the other. Place the other hand on the upper part of the front leg. Pull shoulder blade back and then pull tubing to abdominals. Hold and repeat.

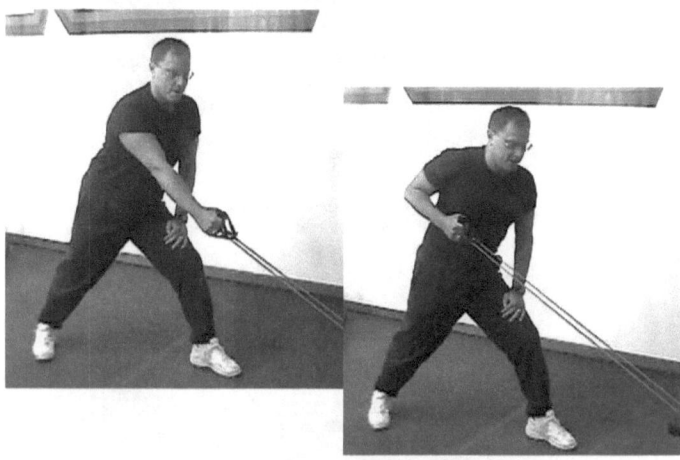

Exercise can be performed with low pulley as well using same directions.

INTERNAL SHOULDER ROTATION

Internal Shoulder Rotation will develop strength and range of motion in the shoulder joint. This movement uses the Latissimus Dorsi, Teres Major and the Subscapularis.

When performing this movement, anchor the tubing above your head and face away from the anchor. Hold the tubing handle in one hand your upper arm at shoulder level. Bend elbow to 90 degrees. Without moving elbow, slowly rotate your shoulder until your forearm is parallel to the floor. Hold and return to start position.

SPECIAL INSTRUCTIONS: It is very important to keep your upper arm parallel to floor.

CAUTION: TUBES AND BANDS MAY BREAK. FOR SAFETY REASONS ALLOW TUBES AND BANDS TO REACH ROOM TEMPERATURE AND ALWAYS CHECK FOR WEAR BEFORE EXERCISING

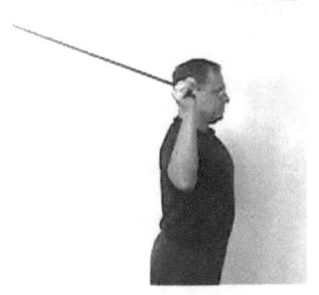
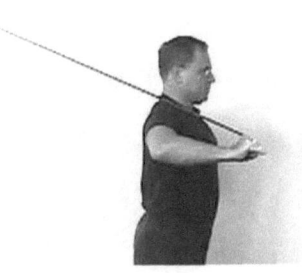

ABDOMINAL CRUNCH WITH LATERAL FLEXION

The Abdominals are important in maintaining posture and providing back stability. The abdominal muscles, when contracted, will relax the middle and upper back muscles. Performing this movement works the Rectus Abdominus, Internal and External Obliques and Transverse Abdominus.

When performing this movement, lie on your back on the floor or a bench. Place feet up on bench or chair and pull your knees back so they are over your belt line. Tuck your chin (press back of neck down to surface), gently press heels down against bench or chair. Slowly curl your upper torso, bringing your shoulders towards your knees keeping your chin tucked and the lower back in contact with the surface. Hold and slowly bring your shoulder toward your hip. Return to center. Hold and slowly lower until shoulders contact surface and repeat.

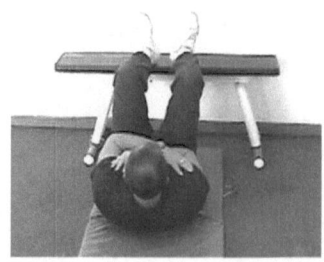 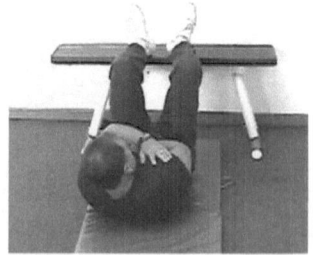

HORIZONTAL BILATERAL SHOULDER ABDUCTION

The Horizontal Bilateral Shoulder Abduction Exercise will strengthen the posterior shoulder muscles while relaxing the chest and anterior shoulder muscles. Performing this movement will turn on the Posterior Deltoid, and Rhomboids muscles while turning off the Pectorals.

When performing this movement, secure tubing at shoulder level. Stand facing the secured tube. Hold handles in both hands and directly in front of mid chest. With hands at chest level, with elbow slightly bent, pull shoulder blades together and pull tubing away from secured end until arms are straight out to side. Reps are to be performed in a slow, controlled manner.

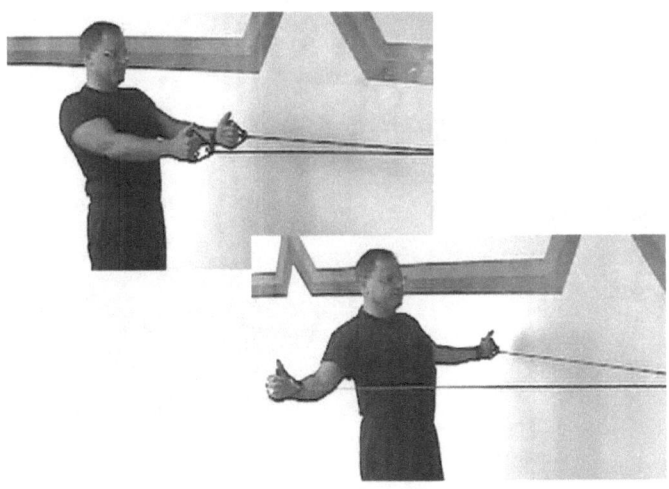

DORSIFLEXION

Dorsiflexion will build the Anterior Tibialis group while relaxing the muscles of the calf.
When performing this movement, Stand up straight with feet at approximately shoulder with apart; pull the top of the foot toward your body or "toes to nose". Hold and return to start position. If you have a problem with balance when in the toe up position, you may want to hold on to something to help maintain proper form throughout the exercise.
SPECIAL INSTRUCTIONS: Add Terminal Flicks at the end of set when ready.

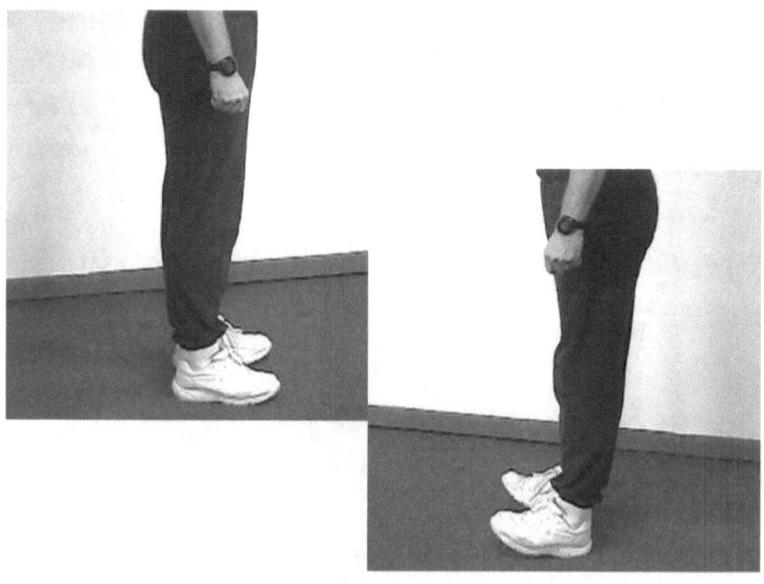

EXERCISE AND THE LYMPHATIC SYSTEM

Exercise has many benefits. It increases metabolism, tones muscles, improves circulation and joint range of motion (ROM). Whether you're running, walking, lifting weights or cycling, muscles are contracting and relaxing. Those muscle contractions might just be accomplishing more than you think.

You may or may not have heard of peripheral heart action (PHA), but PHA may be the most important reason to exercise. When a muscle contracts, blood is trapped within the muscle where the oxygen in the blood is quickly used up to convert glycogen into the energy needed for the muscle to contract. When the muscle relaxes, the venous blood is released carrying toxins and acid away and newly oxygenated blood flushed into the muscle.

It is the very act of muscle contractile and relaxation that make up PHA. For example, if a soldier stands at attention for too long, he will eventually pass out. Why? Because, the heart isn't designed to pump blood efficiently through the body alone—it requires muscle movement. Without movement it is difficult for the venous blood to release its toxins into the lymphatic system to ultimately exit in urine and perspiration.

What is the lymphatic system? Lymph is a clear fluid that rids the body of toxins. Dead cells, fat, viruses and particles of undigested food that seep through the stomach wall, to name a few, are carried away by lymph. With T- and B-Lymphocytes, lymph is one of the first lines of defense for the immune system. The most common example of lymph cleansing is the common cold. Your lymphatic system is hard at work keeping you immune from toxins and disease.

By now you're probably wondering what this all has to do with exercise. More than you would think. By way of muscle contractile, the valves in the lymphatic system open and close allowing the lymph fluid to move the toxins through the body and eventually exiting through perspiration and urine.

One of the most popular methods of lymphatic health exercises is rebounding. By bouncing up and down on a rebounder the fluids are pushed against the one way valves that are placed throughout the lymphatic system. When these valves open they allow the lymph fluid into the next chamber. Then as the muscles relax, the valves close until the next contraction.

It's Not Too Late!

Nearly all exercise helps to move lymph fluid as it travels through the body, but rebounding has been considered the most effective by far. There is another way. An effective and well thought out circuit training regime can give you great benefits in regards to lymphatic flow as well as cardiovascular fitness.

Developed by Dr. Robert Gajda, a former body building champion, The PHA exercise system can answer all your fitness needs: strength and conditioning, cardiovascular fitness and lymphatic exercise. **The PHA is designed for the more experienced exerciser and should be used with caution. If you feel any pain or become light headed, stop immediately and call your physician.**

The system is based on sequencing multiple sets of three to four exercises per sequence. Each sequence starts with a primary exercise, (some examples: squat, bench presses, leg presses, jumps, military press), a secondary exercise, (some examples: lat pulls, rows leg extensions, hamstring curls, hip extensions), a recovery exercise (abdominals, low back, calves, tibialis) and isolation exercise (biceps, triceps).

Perform each sequence in order then repeat one or two times depending on how many sets you want to perform before continuing on to the next sequence. (I recommend starting with one or two sets of each sequence and no more than four sequences per workout). Perform no fewer than 10 and no more than 15 repetitions per movement. As your body adjusts to the system, you will be able to work in any rep range needed depending on whet your goal is.

Sample sequences:

Squats, Lat Pull, Spinal Extensions, Shoulder Extensions

Bench Press, Low Spinal Extensions, Calf Raises, Shoulder Adduction

Leg Press, Seated Rows, Abdominal Crunch, shoulder Hyperflexion,

Push-ups, Leg Extensions, Dorsiflexion, Shoulder Abduction

Along with the terrific health benefits that can be derived from using a PHA, this system can bring a welcomed change when you're looking to spice up your program.

Remember, the sky is the limit. With a little imagination, peripheral heart action can take your workouts to the next level. **Always check with your doctor before starting this, or any exercise program.**

SECTION THREE

SHOULDER STABILIZATION

How do you prevent that shoulder injury? Traditional shoulder exercises, such as overhead presses and lateral raises don't target the muscles that make up the rotator-cuff, only the prime movers; anterior and lateral deltoids. The rotator-cuff is made up of four separate muscles that wrap around the shoulder joint for internal, external and lateral rotation and stabilization. Overuse or using too much weight on shoulder exercises can cause the tendons to the rotator muscles to become inflamed and painful. Proper shoulder stabilization can help to prevent this

But how do we stabilize the shoulders? This can be accomplished by using the shoulder girdle muscles. Let's look at the rhomboids. The rhomboids main function is to glide the scapulae over the ribcage toward the midline of the body. By contracting these muscles (squeeze your shoulder blades together and down before performing the movement) the scapulae are pulled back retracting the shoulders. By using this simple movement while performing shoulder work you will stabilize the rotator-cuff and the AC (shoulder) joint protecting them from injury.

The scapular retraction will also make any upper body movement more effective: bench press, lat pull, shoulder press, flies, you name it. This simple move can increase productivity and safety to the shoulder muscles and rotator-cuff.

PLAY BALL

So, you think you can still throw some leather and swing the bat. Sure it's been twenty years (or more) since you won that shiny trophy, but the idea of joining a Masters Baseball team just keeps rattling around in your head.

Twenty years is a long time, especially when it comes to sports. As we age, joints stiffen and we get a little thicker around the middle. If you aren't in an exercise program, I suggest that you get to the gym and start one. A little conditioning will go a long way to help you achieve your goal. Even if you are in an exercise program, chances are pretty good that you haven't stayed in baseball condition. For those of you who are intent lacing up the spikes again there are ways to still get into baseball shape.

First of all, I must caution you—take it slow. Don't jump right in with both feet. Remember, it's been a long time since you've played the game. Even MLB players start spring training out slowly. This article will focus on training for three main facets of the game: throwing, hitting and running.

Let's start with throwing. Throwing is a shoulder motion pretty much reliant on a set of four muscles called the rotator cuff. This group of muscles dictates, what in baseball is called the arm slot. External rotation pulls the arm back, internal rotation flings the ball and two lateral rotators handle the braking action so the shoulder isn't pulled out when the ball is thrown.

A sensible weight training program is essential in strengthening the shoulders and upper torso. Start with light weights and progress as your strength level allows. Try the reverse fly and shoulder extension exercises.

Start some light throwing with the short toss. As your arm feels more comfortable with the movement, still throwing lightly, increase the throwing distance. After a few sessions, when your arm adjusts to the distance, start throwing a little harder. In all cases stop before your shoulder is fatigued so it won't be sore for the next session.

Hitting a round ball with a round bat is one of the most difficult, if not the most difficult, tasks in sports. It is a complex combination of shoulders, midsection and hips. During the swing, the hands cannot get to far in front or behind the hips so it is very important for the hips to turn into the ball. One way to train is to practice swinging into a heavy punching bag. (Wrapping duct tape around the center of the bag should reinforce the vinyl enough to keep it from splitting.) This will help you time your swing so your hands and hips move together.

The next step would be to hit off a tee. Yes, I said a tee. If it's good enough for the pro's I think it's good enough for you. Use an adjustable tee so you can practice hitting high and low. Then, when you feel comfortable with your swing, head for the nearest batting cage before hitting live pitching. If you've been neglecting the midsection it's time to get to work. Crunches are a great way to start, but make sure that you perform some core exercises that include torso rotation.

In baseball the only time you jog is out to your position. To run the bases or make that spectacular catch in the gap you have to sprint. If you're already a distance runner, you're almost there. The difference is, sprinting is not aerobic (with oxygen), its anaerobic (without oxygen) much like lifting weights. If you don't run, this would be a good time to start.

Try running three times a week. Start out with five minutes and try to increase your time every week. Once you feel comfortable add a 6 to 10 second sprint (running as fast as you can) sometime during each run increasing it to two to three sprints per session. Remember, sprinting is an explosive, anaerobic exercise, so weight training would be extremely beneficial. I recommend squats and lunges to strengthen the lower extremities.

Always warm up properly before starting

any exercise; this includes hitting and throwing sessions. A brisk five minute walk or jog will suffice. You're not as young as you were the last time you played so a little caution goes a long way. After three to five weeks of training, I think you'll be ready to lace them up and relive the 'glory days'. Good luck!

FIVE TIPS TO BETTER GOLF

With spring always just around the corner it's time to get ready for what has become America's favorite activity... Golf. Yes friends it's time to dust off those mighty clubs and head to the mall for the newest high-tech equipment designed to improve your game.

There *is* one piece of equipment that shouldn't be neglected... You! Golf is a sport that the human body was not specifically designed to perform. So, let's take a look at some tips that will ease the stress that golf can put on your body and that just might improve your score.

Let's look at balance. All sports performance is based on balance and how the body will act and react as it is hurtling through time and space. The mid-course correction muscles help keep the body stabilized throughout the swing. They compensate as the weight shifts from the swing phase into the follow through. What keeps your body from falling forward or the direction of the swing? Balance! If you improve your balance you will be far more stable during your swing.

One simple way to improve balance is the one-foot stand. Try standing nice and straight with feet at about shoulder width apart. Keep your shoulders pulled back and the abdominals tight. Lift one foot off the floor and hold it slightly out in front. Hold this position as long as you can. Your goal is to be able to stand without wobbling for about thirty seconds. Switch feet and repeat. If this becomes too easy, check with your local sporting goods store for equipment such as air filled pillows and balance boards that can take you to the next level.

Core strength—here's one that I can't stress enough. The core is made up of the abdominal muscle groups and the muscles of the lower back. These muscles are pretty much what hold us together. Any swinging movement of the upper torso, such as the golf swing, is powered by a series of muscles turning on as others turn off. The stronger your midsection is, the more powerful your swing will be resulting in longer drives without over swinging.

Try two sets of crunches three times per week. Lie on your back with your feet up on a chair or bench so your knees are over your belt line. Tuck your chin and place your arms across your chest. Slowly raise your shoulders toward your knees as you press down lightly on the bench with your heels then return to the starting position. Do as many repetitions as you can. Work up to fifteen repetitions per set. When it gets to easy slow down to four counts up and four counts down.

Now let's work on your rotational joints. When the body performs a function, whether everyday or sport, the joints move in a series of rotations and diagonal angles. One of the problems with the way most people exercise is that they go to the gym and work out on machines that put you in the best mechanical advantage to perform the exercises. This will make you stronger but only in the linear direction and plane that the machine moves in. There is little or no rotation except for the machines that are designed specifically to rotate. But even these do not offer the stabilization training needed in golf.

Don't give up your membership at the YMCA just yet. Take a look around the workout area; my guess is that there are free weights, pulley machines or exercise tubes. Ask one of the attendants or trainers for assistance. They should be able to show you how to use this type of equipment. Most sports stores carry the tubing. It's inexpensive and portable.

Do you need to warm up? Absolutely! The body performs better when the body's core is warmer making the muscles and joints looser and less prone to injury. Warming up is easy. Before you head for the first tee take a brisk five to ten minute walk around the club before you start your ritualistic twists and stretching. It works!

Now that I've brought up stretching I can't stress the dangers of overstretching enough. Light stretching is a great way to loosen up before you start to play. The problem is that just as everything else in America everyone thinks that more is better so when they stretch they twist and force themselves into positions that quite frankly the body doesn't like. For instance; the standing toe touch is dangerous and can injure the lower back, but for some reason people continue to do them. Believe me, your toes are there you don't have to touch them to make sure. When you stretch, and it causes pain, you're hurting yourself.

So please be careful when stretching or performing any exercises and if possible consult a fitness professional to show you the proper techniques.

Fore!

FITNESS WITH CHILDREN AND GRANDCHILDREN

Kids. One day you're standing over their crib, the next your attending their college graduation. Anyone could understand a parent (boomers are still having families) or grandparent's reluctance in missing one moment of a child's life much less a myriad of hours running in place on a treadmill.

Former U.S. Surgeon General, Dr. C. Everett Koop said, "A survey conducted by Shape Up America has revealed that child care responsibilities are interfering with the efforts of many families to get more exercise and at the same time we know that many children are now overweight or obese. The solution is a commitment on the part of the entire family to spend more time together; that includes too grandparents too. The former Surgeon General also added, "The pleasure of your company is the best reward a child can receive and the best gift that you can give."

Even as schools continue to drop physical education classes in favor of more academics, (According to The American Obesity Association, 78% of parents in the U.S. believe that physical education or recess should not be reduced or replaced with academic classes.) child obesity continues to grow.

Kids aren't the only Americans dealing with weight related health issues. Parents need to take a look at some statistics as well. In the latest data from the National Center for Health, 30% of adults, 20 years and older suffer from obesity—that's over 60 million people!

Getting Started.

There are ways for you to combat these astonishing figures—together as a family. But where do you start? The first thing to do is set up regularly scheduled times during each week for family physical activity. Once this is done, have each member of the family come up with a group activity. Try to make the activities such that all family members can perform. You want everyone to succeed.

Decide whether your activities will take place at home or whether your family wants to join a health club or community center. I see parents and grandparents going to the gym with their kids and grandchildren. Swimming is a fun family activity and most communities have an indoor public pool available for year round use. Group exercise classes, such as step or spinning can be fun for the whole family. Beginning exercise classes are usually able to accommodate most age groups. Check with your local Park District or YMCA for more information about family memberships and programs.

Exercising At Home

If you should decide that keeping everyone at home, especially with little ones, your activities will make consistent participation more convenient. There are plenty of tips for successful fitness. First, designate specific areas in the home, indoor and outdoor, where physical activity is to take place. Designating specific places for activity gives the family a similar sense of purpose as going to the gym, or health club. Make sure the area is safe for whatever activities the family chooses (especially if Grandpa is clumsy). Who knows, you may find yourself climbing, jumping or rolling and you don't want anyone getting injured. Be aware of your surroundings, I recommend an area with a high ceiling. And remember, you should always consult your family physician before starting any type of exercise program. Safety first!

It's Not Too Late!

There are many tools available for in-home family fitness. If the children are high school age, you can install a home gym for lifting weights. There are many multi-gyms on the market today that as many as three family members can use at the same time.

For families with younger children, simple calisthenics using body weight is safe and effective for increasing fitness levels. Push-ups, abdominal crunches, standing trunk rotations, arm rotations, walking or running in place are only a few of the exercises that can be performed in a limited amount of space. As your family progresses, try light hand or ankle weights to increase the difficulty level. Remember to always start with lighter weights, slowly progressing as everybody adapts.

If you have a little more space then there are many tools available to help with your program as near as the local Sporting goods store. Fitness or resistance balls (Most brands come with exercise suggestions and safe programs for beginners.) If you're looking for a great cardiovascular activity, try jumping rope. It might sound easy but believe me it's not! Jumping rope provides not only a great workout but also helps in developing motor skills needed in many sports. Another great group activity is step aerobics. Steps and risers are available at most sporting good stores and are easy to assemble Create your own step classes with the instructions that come with the equipment or purchase one of the many step videos that are currently on the market. Once the whole family has the hang of it, you can all take turns in leading the group.

Adding an exercise bike, treadmill or elliptical machines to your in-home exercise arsenal can add another dimension to your family workouts. Not only can each member use it individually to enhance their fitness program, but these machines can also be incorporated into the group routine by having one less station for exercises and rotating each family member onto the machine as the others go through the routine. Set a time limit then switch. This is a great way to break things up.

One of the more popular in-home exercise devises is the mini tram. This tiny, round trampoline has been on the exercise scene forever and still supplies one of the best, jumping or running in place, workouts. Nominally priced in most sporting good and department stores, the mini tram can provide hours of exercise and fun for the entire family. One little tip, wherever you perform mini tram exercises, make sure that it has a fairly high ceiling. If you're not careful, a little too much bounce could result in a bad bump on the head or worse. Remember—always—safety first!

If you have trouble developing programs that work for your family, the internet is a wonderful resource for fitness programs. Your local bookstore has hundreds of exercise books and videos for all ages. Another option is to hire a personal trainer to design a program that will work for your family. Most training companies have programs that will fit your needs. Be sure to check all trainer certifications to insure that he or she is qualified and experienced enough to work with you and your grand/children.

Going Outdoors

Family walks and bicycle rides can be fun way to enhance your fitness. Keep a log to track the miles and pace so your family can measure their progress. Modified sports are a great way to keep the family off the couch and out into the fresh air. Have fun modifying kick ball, softball, basketball or even football to fit your family size and children's ages. Be creative but keep everybody moving as much as possible.

Get Involved

Take the time to speak with the children's physical education teacher. They can give you insight into what type of activities children participate in at school as well as how you can provide support. Be aware of changes in curriculum. Many schools are restricting or eliminating physical education. Be proactive. Contact the local school board to prevent this from happening at your school.

Busy Baby Boomers also need to be aware of other fitness opportunities. Take a walk after lunch. Use the stairs instead of the elevator. Speak to your employer about providing incentives to employees who participate in a regular fitness program or possibly establishing one in the workplace.

Use your imagination. Fitness can be fun for the whole family. What better way is there to spend quality time with children then doing something that will benefit theirs and your health and well being? So come on—you, the kids and the grandkids—get off that couch and build some muscles and some wonderful memories along the way.

IN CLOSING

Please keep in mind that no book on exercise, no matter who may produce it, is a good substitute for working with a trained fitness professional. All I have attempted to do, I hope successfully, in this book is to give the reader a little better understanding of what good logical fitness training is all about.

In the near future there will be additional booklets available that will

It's Not Too Late!

compliment and help you progress to an even higher level of fitness. Other future booklets will involve specific joint, core and circuit training programs. These will be available in mail order only. For more information e-mail us at tfcon@comcast.net

GET YOUR MIND SET...
CONFIDENCE WILL LEAD YOU!